A WOMAN'S TRUTH™

A life truly worth living.

Priceless teachings reveal your transformational
journey ahead. Obstacles to self-care are explored
as clear and loving intentions are conceived.

Please note:

The written or spoken information, ideas, procedures and suggestions contained and presented in 'A WOMAN'S TRUTH' workshops and books are meant for educational purposes only and are not for diagnosis. It should not be used as a substitute for your physician's advice. 'A WOMAN'S TRUTH' is not therapy and is not intended to replace the recommendations of a licensed health practitioner. It is the responsibility of the reader to consult with their own medical Doctor, Counselor, Therapist or other competent professional regarding any condition before adopting any of the suggestions in this book.

A WOMAN'S TRUTH™

*Dedicated to the Divine essence
of the feminine who resides within us all.*

MISSION STATEMENT

To guide and facilitate women
in becoming their most beautiful and radiant selves.

To acknowledge and embrace the well of love
and power which lies within all women and to ignite the
awakening and embodying of this life force.

To empower each woman, through exquisite self-care and love,
to live her fullest life possible, and to walk her path of wisdom
and truth, as she shares this light and knowledge
with all beings.

IN DEEP GRATITUDE

Thank you

The creation, birth and life of 'A Woman's Truth' would not have been possible without the love, support and devotion from the following angels in my life:

My beautiful daughter Megan who naturally embodies the teachings of living in her truth and integrity, thank you for the creative gift of the beautiful artwork. Helena Nelson-Reed for her generosity of spirit in allowing her extraordinary artwork, which embodies the teachings so magnificently, to grace the covers. Dennise Marie Keller for her unwavering support and dedication to the teachings and for proofing, editing, aligning and translating my vision into the technical world of manifestation. Dan Fowler for his creative genius and dedication. Lucy Alexander and Suzanne Ryan, my dearest friends for their amazing editing and wholehearted encouragement. Monica Marsh for her commitment, support and belief in the workshops. Maggie Crawford, my mum, for her proofing and for being a living example of the teachings. Cait Myer and Katie Steen for their patience and ability to decipher my handwriting and for formatting the books. Bethany Kelly for her support. Deborah Waring for holding the space for the conception of 'A Woman's Truth' to be born and for her insight in the first year of teaching and Emmanuel for believing in my vision.

My mentors and teachers Rod Stryker, Adyashanti and Alison Armstrong, Max Simon and Jeffrey Van Dyk for their continuous and guiding light in my life, their never-ending belief in my potential and for always teaching me the way to evolve into my highest and most potent self. And to all of you beautiful and courageous women who are committing to living your truth and transforming into your most radiant selves,

thank you.

A PRELUDE

An Overture to A Woman's Truth.

*I*n the world today there appears to be an energetic movement towards expanded consciousness and awareness. Never before has the truth wanted to burst through the shell and into the light as powerfully as it does right now. The spirit of the time is urging us to expand into more layers of ourselves and to prepare us for a future in which authenticity is vital.

We can no longer be satisfied with 'almost' living. We can no longer, be fine with 'kind of' doing the right thing for ourselves and others, and we can no longer ignore the inner wisdom that guides us towards our right path in life. The truth is beckoning us to step into its light, and Miranda's 'Woman's Truth' work is an important part of this movement.

Miranda is one of the wise women of our time.

She has devoted her life to guide women and men gently through the challenges we face and to show an enlightened way of thinking and living. By being a source of wisdom to the people around her, and by manifesting her visions and sharing them, she is a gift of great beauty to this world.

Miranda has created not only this book, but also a whole body of work that can transform the lives of women by showing them how to take care of their body, their mind and their spirit. That is what is so unique and lovely about this particular work! Miranda manages to manifest great spiritual truth in practical doing.

Starting from the basics of sleep, nutrition and movement and moving up through the layers of our beings, Miranda teaches women how to take loving leadership of their lives. Originating from the deep insight that we cannot live our life to its fullest without integrating all areas of ourselves into every part of our daily life, this book shows us how to make choices as a whole being.

When we take charge of our life, when we dare to face what is no longer serving us and clean out the old to make space for the new, positive change is inevitable. When a person changes, she forces the environment around her to also change and the ripple effect is great. I am grateful and honored to have experienced the Woman's Truth work, and to know Miranda. This book has the power to transform the lives of many women, and thereby families and communities around the world.

~ **Birla Angelica Hood**

A WOMAN'S TRUTH™

Gems of Truth

A DAILY PRACTICE

commit to yourself

*F*ollow these simple steps daily as a way to instill and strengthen your heartfelt resolve to love yourself. This will help to keep you aligned, transforming and on track, giving you a stable foundation for the rest of your life. As a gift to yourself, please mark the teachings as you read them through and congratulate yourself with each one. See each day as a commitment to take exquisite care of yourself.

A LIFE WORTH LIVING

"Never give from your well.
Always give from your overflow."
~ Rumi

All too often as women, your own needs are denied for the benefit of others as you orchestrate your life through demands and expectations you feel responsible for. Unfortunately, this can leave you without the juice and energy needed to be present fully and to enjoy life. During these readings, you will continually discover more about who you truly are and learn the tools needed to live your most authentic and fulfilling life possible. From this place, you will experience being 'full to overflowing' and all the joy and energy this brings.

As you delve into these teachings, you will explore, laugh, study, share, and freely express who you are. In this sacred space, you will ultimately learn your truth as a woman in order to shine, to embody your own beauty, believe in your own worth, and take exquisite care of yourself. For only in this way can you truly be of service.

During these guidebooks, many of the basic needs of women will be explored such as sleep, nutrition, creativity, movement and time to replenish. A topic has been chosen for each book and a cohesive and practical foundation is laid out to inspire and guide you. This will bring about a new strength and resolve which will allow your needs to become a priority, without letting your outer world dictate otherwise. By the end of our time together, the concept of being confident, loving, serene and passionate will no longer be a distant fantasy. Instead, these and many other extraordinary qualities that you naturally embody as a woman will flow with ease, grace and love.

With life's demands so high, it has become imperative that your needs are first acknowledged, honored and then taken care of. From this vantage point, your relationship with yourself then has the potential to be transformed into one of self-love. The beauty is this in turn creates a life that not only fulfills you and your life's purpose, but also allows everyone touched by your presence to receive this gift.

I look forward to spending this precious time with you.

Welcome to A Woman's Truth.

Sincerely and with love,

Miranda

LIVING YOUR TRUTH

One step at a time.

The teachings of 'A Woman's Truth' are a heartfelt commitment to falling deeply back in love with yourself. As you learn to trust in taking care of yourself and prioritizing your needs as vital and responsible, a priceless gift is unveiled allowing you to shine your brilliance onto the world. The following is the path you will be walking with 'A Woman's Truth'. You may notice how some of the teachings and simple practices will resonate more with you than others. This is natural, yet interestingly the ones you want to avoid may well be the weak link in the chain of your life that on some level will serve you to strengthen. Each layer of 'A Woman's Truth' builds upon itself, resulting in a strong foundation for the rest of your life.

A Woman's Truth

A life truly worth living.

Priceless teachings reveal your transformational
journey ahead. Obstacles to self-care are explored
as clear and loving intentions are conceived.

The Grandeur of Sleep

Permission to rest.

Miraculous benefits are realized as the worlds of sleep,
relaxation and rejuvenation are explored and deeply honored.

Nourishing Nutrition
Reclaim your health and vitality.

Reap the bountiful rewards while eating as nature intended.
Claim your health and vitality with these simple,
yet powerful tools to nourish and heal your body.

Embodying Movement
Ground your whole being.

Restore balance in your life. Discover how to embrace
your whole being through the life-enhancing benefits of body movement.

Body Care
Cherish your body as a temple.

Learn to honor your extraordinary body
as a living temple and listen to the healing messages she whispers.

Feminine Power
Fully access your supreme birthright.

Welcome and reclaim this intrinsic privilege while living
in harmonious balance between the masculine and the feminine.

The Abundance of Wealth
Receive the gifts of prosperity.

Understand the energy flow of prosperity and weave
the threads of abundance throughout the tapestry of your life.

Find Your Authentic Voice
The courage to express who you truly are.

Your greatest ally is born
when you courageously speak your truth and claim your unique power.

Loving Yourself
A love affair with the self.

As you become highly attuned to your own needs,
allow love to lead the way. Grant yourself permission
to honor and express your heart's truest desires.
Love yourself, no matter what.

Living A Spiritual Life
Ground your divine essence here on earth.

Discover what spirituality means to you, by consciously
living between the two worlds of the sacred and the mundane.

Service As A Way Of Life
Ignite the fire of love to truly be of service.

By utilizing the gems of exquisite self-care
on a daily basis and honoring your truth, your mission of service is born.

The Crowning Glory
Fully Rejoice in Being You.

A celebration overflowing with love,
blessings, grace and gratitude. Stand confident within
your truth as your mind begins to serve your heart.

Every time you make a commitment to your own self-care, self-love and self-respect and then follow through, you build trust in yourself. Imagine having a friend who never lets you down. You become your very best advocate, a knight in shining armor, who will always make a stand for you. As you build trust in yourself, your ability to expand your vision and fully live in your magnificence is amplified. This is the heart felt promise you are making to yourself as you walk the path of 'A Woman's Truth'.

THE JOURNEY AHEAD
practice is the path.

Whenever you choose to commit your time, your energy or your money, it is important to know what you are getting in return for your investment. 'A Women's Truth' is orchestrated in such a way for you to receive an abundant reward. Through succinct guidance, clearly laid out information, and a safe and nurturing environment, you will be led down a path of self-discovery.

No two women's journeys are alike, yet the result of making space for whom you truly are and living by this truth is consistent. The moments spent in inquiry are priceless, yet much of the transformation happens during daily life, as you begin to embody the teachings.

Each book clearly describes and reflects the essence of self-love and self-care, which is the foundation of 'A Woman's Truth'. It is therefore vital for you to read, absorb and reflect on the information given to you. This is an invitation for you to deepen the teachings and experiences.

It is highly recommended that you read a page or so a day. This will allow you to absorb the guidance more fully before moving on. A daily connection helps keep the contents alive and your choices and behaviors conscious. As you steep your being in the concepts and teachings, answer the questions and explore the simple, yet poignant exercises, you will gain insights into which of your habits and choices are serving you, and which ones are better released.

One of the reasons these guidebooks are offered one at a time is to give you a feeling of space in your own life, which allows each topic to be clearly defined, taught and explored. Then the teachings can be fully lived through, experienced and absorbed into your daily life. This ample length of time also gives you the chance to melt away any obstacles in your path, so you can become the vibrant being that you already are.

◆ Be patient and loving with yourself on this adventure.

◆ Take time and release all judgment regarding where you *think* you *should* be. This is your journey, your life.

◆ As you become your own advocate and your own steward, your life will beautifully transform.

DISTILL YOUR LIFE
The story versus the point.

Release the story and the truth will be revealed.
Release the past and the present will reveal itself.
Embrace the future and walk through your fears.
Dig out the weeds and the flowers will blossom.
Speak your Truth and your life will become manifest.

As you embark upon this journey, it is vital to reveal what may be limiting your fullest potential. One of the biggest obstacles can be *the story* surrounding certain issues. You may have noticed how attached to the tale you can become and the impact the past is still having on you. It seems the more the story is embellished and built, the more engrained and rooted it can become. Often the core issue or nugget, which is *the point,* is lost in the depths of the details.

Unfortunately, when the story takes over it can become your reality. It can grip your heart and limit your ability to love. It can hold you in past fears. It is then fed like a monster who dictates who you truly are. Just as with any brilliant storyteller, you get lost in the fantasy identify and believe the story to be real. Yet as you unravel the illusion and step back, you begin to realize it may not be the whole truth. You then have the space, like a bird on the wing, to look down and observe fiction from fact.

WHEN YOU ARE ABOUT TO LAUNCH INTO A STORY, ASK YOURSELF THE FOLLOWING QUESTIONS:

◆ What is the heart of the fable that needs to be addressed and nurtured?

◆ What are the few words that would distil this huge dissertation?

◆ What is the point, the truth, the gem that once dug through and revealed, will shine and light your way forward?

Unless you deliver the gold from the dross, you will carry the debris and waste around with you forever. This will weigh you down, block your insight and absorb your energy. As you release the story, the light of your true being will no longer allow a casting of shadows past.

WHO IS SHE?

The self within the self.

Who is the Self that resides in all beings?
Who is the infinite light that shines
Even when we unconsciously choose to dim her brilliance?

Who is the Self who knows without reason the journey ahead?
Who is she that can love and forgive
Even when a situation demands justice and retribution?

Who is she that lives within us all?

Who is this Goddess who would choose love over hate,
Compassion over judgment
And forgiveness over punishment?

Who is she that breathes the pulse of life
And invokes the spark of creation?

Who is she who nurtures and holds in loving arms?
Whose essence can melt away fear?

Who is she, we ask? Who is she?

And as we choose to call her by name
Her essence and being will rise from the ashes.

She is the Self that lives and breathes within you.
She is the Self without the façade of fear and lies.

She is who you came here to be.
She is your birthright.
She is who will be birthed and lived
As you fall madly and deeply in love with yourself.
She already is.
She is you.

THIS IS YOUR LIFE
cultivate a relationship with yourself.

The foundation of 'A Woman's Truth' is ultimately about becoming increasingly aware of your own intimate relationship with yourself. As your life progresses you will become more and more awake to what you need on a daily basis. Your focus will no longer be limited to merely functioning, but will shift and expand, so you can clearly see what will be required for you to thrive. As you consciously choose to give yourself the gifts of self-care, they become an integral part of your rhythm and the vital tools that you will tap into for the rest of your life.

This guidebook focuses on self-inquiry and turning inward. You will become aware of your lifestyle choices that are helping you or others which may be hindering you.

change can only begin with awareness.

Therefore, unless you question and inquire, it might not be obvious how a shift in behavior is needed. As women, some of our ingrained behaviors have been passed down through the generations. Have you ever wondered why sometimes you may be acting out of character, yet it feels strangely familiar to act that way? What is taught by our ancestors can often become an automatic response to certain situations. Therefore, it is vital to pause long enough to discern how you are reacting is in alignment with your true nature. It seems as though at this pivotal point in the history of women, we now have the freedom to choose differently, if it is appropriate.

"While I was at boarding school in England, we were given a choice to sleep in or eat breakfast. Because breakfast consisted of the same white tasteless bread we had for tea, I chose, for seven years, to sleep in. Over this time, I formed the habit of not eating breakfast and I was never hungry in the morning. Years later, when I started to study nutrition, I kept on hearing how breakfast is the most important meal of the day. I began to question my strongly held conviction 'I don't eat breakfast'. Once I realized that I could eat whatever I wanted, the act of breaking my night time fast and nourishing my body now became a conscious choice each morning." ~ Miranda

During the journey of 'A Woman's Truth', a loving structure is built surrounding the care of the physical form. This is called 'The Foundational Trinity'. The body will trigger an instinctive stress reaction, unless its basic survival needs are taken care of. By honoring and responding to your natural and essential requirements for sleep, food, water and movement, you will rise out of the realm of survival into the world of fulfillment.

In the 'The Grandeur Of Sleep' deep relaxation and rest is explored. Time is dedicated to the necessity of sleep and its extraordinary healing abilities. In this highly-strung, hyperactive and technologically driven world, the concept of becoming still, quiet and relaxed is often neglected and not readily accessible, let alone received. Moreover, as you know, a well-rested woman is a beautiful thing.

As your sleep life is stabilized, the world of 'Nourishing Nutrition' is explored, including the impact food and water has on your life. It is not always about what you eat and drink that can cause issues. Rather it can be about what you are not eating and drinking, for which the body is desperately craving! It is much easier to add the good stuff, little by little, rather than harshly deprive yourself making your emotions take over and the resolve to eat well is discarded after only a few days.

Miranda's food bible 'The Versatile Vegetable' from her 'The Food of Life' series is a valuable asset. This book will outline the essential ingredients for a healthy, energized and vital life.

'Embodying Movement' explores the gifts that moving the body give you and how exercise will ground your body and increase your energy supply. A sedentary life style can greatly impede the body's ability to remain young, vital, strong and healthy. Unfortunately, modern-day living no longer naturally exercises the body. Finding a movement you enjoy and look forward to is the key. Then carving out the precious time to actually explore, play and perform the exercise will allow you to reap all of the movement's benefits.

In 'Body Care', the world of taking care of your skin, your hair and even your toes is explored. Each body part is addressed. Ranging from how to travel and stay well to keeping the sinuses clear. In 'A Woman's Truth', the impetus behind any care and pampering of the self always stems from a demonstration of love.

As you cultivate this loving relationship with yourself, you will also align with listening to the many crucial messages your body is telling you. The chances are, if you listen to the beginning of the whispers you will not have to hear the shouts, which can translate as pain or disease in the body.

Once the realm of the physical form is honored, then the teachings and guidebooks transition into the world of the mind and the emotions. Many of the seeds have already been planted. As your resolve to take loving and exquisite care of yourself grows, the desire to be in your power and speak your truth becomes a natural by-product. As you become balanced and living from your center, the concept of self-care and self-love is a normal occurrence and it will flow seamlessly.

The concept of **'Feminine Power'** is then addressed. As a woman, you have a natural strength living within you, but it often lies dormant. Using 'A Council', the masculine and feminine energies are brought back into balance and partnership. It then becomes vividly clear whether it is the masculine or the feminine that is appropriate to bring forward at any given time. When both aspects are honored, many of life's stresses and conflicts are released.

As your physical, mental and emotional energy systems begin to flow and claim their highest possible level of health, so too will your relationship with **'The Abundance Of Wealth'**. During these precious teachings, many limiting beliefs in regards to money will be dismantled. With the use of powerful exercises, the horizon for prosperity, wealth and abundance is literally blown sky high, in a good way!

In the guidebook **'Find Your Authentic Voice'** saying no when appropriate and speaking your truth becomes second nature.

The 'loving yourself no matter what' concept is magnificently demonstrated in **'Loving Yourself'**. A completely new what level of self-care is embodied as all the threads of 'A Woman's Truth' are pulled together into the tapestry of your life. Any weak links are strengthened and your resolve is empowered and prepared for the rest of the teachings.

The conviction of **'Living A Spiritual Life'** is beautifully orchestrated, as your spiritual side is nurtured, held and replenished. The teachings are not connected to any specific religion, yet the guidebook does invoke a strengthening of your relationship with your spiritual nature in whatever capacity this means to you. For some this may mean time in nature, for others it may be meditating. It is not so much about the practice, but rather how it resonates with you and what impact it has on your wellbeing. If it leaves you calm, grateful and aligned in your center, then you have found a spiritual practice that is perfect for you. The foundation for **'Living a Spiritual Life'** is that any moment can be a spiritual moment, if allowed.

As **'A Woman's Truth'** comes to completion, time is spent exploring your mission and purpose here on earth. In **'Service As A Way Of Life'**, you are ultimately serving yourself first, and from this place of 'full to overflowing' you are then able to truly be of service to others. Many of the survival instincts that may have been leading your decision making in the past will vanish as you take exquisite care of your whole being. It is fascinating to watch how different your perception can be when you are standing in a position of power, with a bird's eye view of the whole. From this vantage point, the answers to your life's purpose can become crystal clear and the juice needed to carry it to fruition is abundant.

The last teaching, which is appropriately titled **'The Crowning Glory'**, is a celebration of who you have become. With all your needs taken care of and your will, mind, body and spirit in alignment, you can truly live a life worth living. As your own sphere of energy calibrates to its highest possible level, this quality then ripples out into the world. Choosing to take beautiful care of yourself, allows for the overflow to be spread out into the world which will support and heal this extraordinary place we call home.

"After writing these books, my life changed dramatically. As each book unfolded, I had to live the teachings. 'Practice what you preach', as the old saying goes or 'walk the talk'. Yet the greatest gift and honor was to watch many already beautiful and extraordinary women blossom into their fullest capacities and highest potential. These teachings seem to have the ability to unravel and release whatever is limiting one's life and to encourage each woman to embody her own magnificence and power. I am deeply grateful to be on this path, to access these teachings and be a guide for others to discover and embody their own inner wisdom and brilliance." ~ Miranda

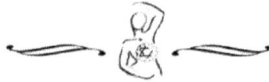

"This is your life, and nobody is going to teach you,
no book, no guru. You have to learn from yourself.
It is an endless thing, it is a fascinating thing and when you learn about
yourself, from yourself, out of that learning wisdom comes.
Then you can live a most extraordinary, happy, beautiful life."
~ Krishnamurti

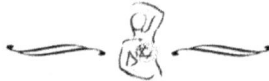

LIVE YOUR DASH
Born 1967 – Died 2062

The question here is are you fully living out your dash or living your life in fear of the date at the end? As the dates of a birth and death are engraved on a headstone, it is worth pondering which is more important: Are these two milestones in time or in actuality, the little dash that depicts your life, the sum of your experiences and your legacy? In hindsight, it seems as though it is all about that dash.

THEREFORE THE NEXT QUESTION TO ASK IS:

◆ Are you fully living out your dash, meaning your life experience?

◆ Are you more concerned with your death or the death of another, that you are not choosing to live your life fully?

◆ What would happen if you lived out each day as though it may be your last?

◆ What would change in your life, and what would you choose to do differently knowing you only had a short time left?

Sometimes when people are diagnosed with a terminal illness, they acknowledge that, along with shock and trauma, they also feel a sense of relief and release. This liberation might allow them to leave the job they have hated for the last ten years or go on their fantasy vacation. It is as if they are receiving permission to live the life of their dreams.

Take a moment to ponder what you would change in your world if you only had a few months to live. This is not about being morbid, but more about imagining how you would spend your precious time, money and energy? You would probably not want to waste it. Rather you would no longer put off all the passions and desires you have been denying yourself.

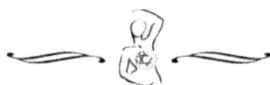

"Death is an advisor
looking over our shoulder,
showing us how to live."
~ Anonymous

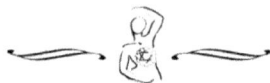

Give yourself this gift and allow that little dash in the middle to become the story of your life in such a way that people talk, books are written and the theme will be:

"She really lived her life!"

16

OBSTACLES TO SELF-CARE

Discover your limiting belief.

No matter what is happening around you, first take care of yourself. When you are balanced in your own relationship, all things will be gradually added to your life and the changes you have asked for will occur. The following is a list of obstacles that may be blockages to taking exquisite and beautiful care of you. This is all about getting to know your dam wall so you can dismantle it slowly and lovingly.

CHOOSE THE OBSTACLES
MOST DETRIMENTAL TO LIVING A HAPPY LIFE:

Please feel free to add any of your own!

◊   Self-care has never been a priority

◊   Not conscious of self-care

◊   Unclear of what self-care means

◊   Not a part of your daily life

◊   Feel unworthy or undeserving

◊   Already feel overwhelmed

◊   Too many other responsibilities

◊   Lack of time, too busy

◊ Cannot afford it

◊ Duty to care for others first

◊ Other relationships take priority

◊ Giving to others relieves guilt

◊ Feel guilty when doing self-care

◊ Procrastination over self-care

◊ Laziness

◊ Lack of willpower

◊ Belief that idleness is the devil's workshop

◊ Undisciplined

◊ Feel too stuck to change

◊ Belief other commitments are more important

◊ Prioritizing other commitments

◊ Prioritizing your work

◊ You can do it all

◊ You do not actually need self-care

◊ Being too flexible

◊ Harsh self-judgment

◊ Needing to be liked

◊ What will others think of you?

◊ Self-sacrifice is rewarded

◊ Self-care is a luxury

◊ Self-care is not important

◊ Being comfortable with discomfort

◊ If you are not productive you are useless

◊ Believing only you can take care of things

◊ Denial that you even have needs

◊ Might miss something

◊ Belief you will rest once it is all done

◊ No role model for self-care

◊ Fear of change

◊ Fear of feeling or being alone

◊ Fear of being a narcissist

◊ Fear of being selfish

- ◊ Fear of self-care causing a conflict with others

- ◊ Fear of repercussions

- ◊ Fear of standing in your power

- ◊ Fear of being too powerful

- ◊ Fear of being passionate

- ◊ Fear of being creative

- ◊ Having a weak relationship with your needs

- ◊ Needing to adapt to other people's needs

- ◊ Not giving yourself permission for self-care

- ◊ Allowing the outside world to dictate what you do

- ◊ Having to be a wonder woman with a to-do list

- ◊ Your sense of self-worth hinges on what you do for others

- ◊ Why stop starving yourself

- ◊ Should be grateful for what you have therefore should not need anything else

- ◊ The feeling of how dare you take care of yourself?

- ◊ Being uncomfortable with the quiet and stillness of no drama

- ◊ You have to be practically dead before you can take care of yourself

◊ You believe you already take enough care of yourself

◊ Reluctance or fear of introspection or looking inward

◊ Resentment that you have to do all this self-care

◊ Which is your weakest link in regards to taking beautiful care of yourself?

  ◊ Physical   ◊ Mental   ◊ Emotional   ◊ Spiritual

◊ Any other obstacles…

GET TO KNOW YOURSELF

"watch your thoughts; they become words.
watch your words; they become actions.
watch your actions; they become habits.
watch your habits; they become your character.
watch your character;
it becomes your destiny."
~ Lao Tzu

The following questionnaire is a way for you to become aware of your daily patterns and habits. Through this inquiry, you will gather the information needed for good healthy behaviors to be strengthened and the others gently laid to rest.

As a human being, we are on a continuous journey of self-discovery and experience. This sacred place you are entering is your internal world, rather than the external environment. It involves the choices you are making in relationship to yourself on a daily basis. These are the behaviors and patterns that may go unnoticed by others, yet will have a huge impact on your wellbeing. Much of your strength as a woman can come from the resolve to replenish and fill your own well and essence first, before taking care of others. This concept of nurturing and prioritizing yourself is often a foreign one, yet it is this premise that is the foundation for 'A Woman's Truth'. This internal questioning will give you insight and clarity into how to treat yourself lovingly.

As you ponder and answer the following questions:

◆ Be Honest.

◆ Breathe.

Let go of any judgment surrounding this inquiry.

PERSONAL HABITS

Each personal habits is a direct reflection
of whether you have love for yourself or not.

Take a few moments to inquire whether your daily routine is adding life force, vitality and health to your life. On the other hand, are your habits harmful, numbing or in some way preventing you from living the fullest possible life? Are you underestimating the value or detriment of a daily routine?

◆ Do you watch TV?

◊ Yes ◊ No

◆ How many hours a day?

◆ Do you use a computer and other electronics?

◊ Yes ◊ No

◆ How many hours a day?

◆ What do you do to distract or de-stress yourself?

- ◊ Watch TV
- ◊ Shop
- ◊ Tidy
- ◊ Clean
- ◊ Read
- ◊ Smoke
- ◊ Exercise
- ◊ Talk
- ◊ Sleep
- ◊ Sit at computer
- ◊ Take drugs
- ◊ Have sex
- ◊ Eat
- ◊ Drink alcohol
- ◊ Move house or redecorate
- ◊ Gossip
- ◊ Play
- ◊ Do them all

◆ What else do you do to release stress in yourself?

◆ What else could you do to release tension?

◆ Do you meditate or pray daily?

- ◊ Yes
- ◊ No

◆ Do you take time for yourself daily? (space just for you)

- ◊ Yes
- ◊ No

◈ Do you have regular check-ups with your doctor?

◊ Yes ◊ No

◈ Do you get regular bodywork such as massages, acupuncture, reflexology, chiropractic or other alternative therapies?

◊ Yes ◊ No

◈ Do you spend time in nature on a regular basis?

◊ Yes ◊ No

◈ Do you have special habits that are nurturing to you?

◊ Yes ◊ No

◈ What are these nurturing habits?

◈ Do you go to therapy, counseling or receive energy work?

◊ Yes ◊ No

◈ Do you tend to complete tasks or leave things half-done?

◊ Yes ◊ No

SETTING INTENTIONS

"Energy follows thought."
~ Albert Einstein

*A*nother way of translating this statement is to realize how your own personal energy bank feeds whatever you are thinking about. Depending on how invested you are in the thought effects how much energy is sent out. Imagine a light bulb. Without any electric current, it is just a piece of glass and metal with a filament. Yet as soon as you plug it into a light socket and flick the electric switch on, the bulb lights up. Your thoughts are no different. The confusion begins when throughout the day; both your conscious and unconscious thoughts are being energized. There are the ones that you know about, yet there is also the gamut of old memories, beliefs and patterns of which you may be unaware. The later could well be having their wicked way with you.

Your thoughts are rather like an iceberg. The conscious ones are the tip that you see above the surface. Yet, below the depths, there are vast quantities of unconscious memories that you do not see, but are ominously present. Some of these unconscious patterns may be wonderfully positive, yet others may be limiting your very existence. Obviously, it is good to know what is what.

Money is always a good illustration. You want to be wealthy and not worry about money. Yet you are being driven by a deeply held, old unconscious belief that you do not deserve to be rich. Unfortunately, it is immaterial how much time you spend consciously thinking you should be prosperous, because your underlying belief of not being worthy is more powerful and will override the conscious thoughts.

Another example is someone who desperately wants a romantic partner. They date, they go on line, yet there is always some glitch. By digging deeper, there is often a subconscious belief that being in an intimate relationship will cause heartache, possibly because of previous experiences. These cellular memories are deeply embedded as a way to attempt to protect you. The fear of pain then outweighs the desire for partnership.

If you are noticing your desires are not coming to fruition, it is time to dive into the unconscious world to discover what other belief may be stronger. It may often be connected to your survival and quite possibly be childlike in nature. This is especially true if you have been wishing for something over a long period of time and it is still eluding you. Most likely, there is an unconscious block. This is why self-inquiry is vital.

A GOOD QUESTION TO ASK IS:

◈ What am I afraid will happen, if this intention becomes a reality?

If you seek wealth, yet you are still only just breaking even, it may mean that fear is driving the situation. For some people, extreme wealth goes against the grain of their ancestral tribe and they believe they will no longer fit in if they become very rich. Another possible fear is that you will no longer be able to gauge if people like you for who you are or just for your money. In addition, greater responsibility can come with abundance and you will no longer be dependent on certain people. For some, staying in the position of the child can feel safer than being accountable to the self. These are just a few possible blockages in the world of money.

Often these beliefs are strongly tied to an old memory, therefore it is vital to trace back to the earliest time you felt the specific feeling or fear.

Then it can be brought to the light, released and set free. As you begin to inquire into your qualms, you can then shed light and awareness on the veil or wall that is surrounding your hearts true desires.

Inquiry will reveal the obstacle.

Remember these old beliefs and patterns are just hiding in your unconscious. You hold the key and can unlock the door at your own pace and at any time. Just by saying an intention and leaving it at that will not necessarily result in an outcome, if there is a stronger, more primal belief behind the scenes.

HOW TO SET AN INTENTION:

◆ **Invoke a deep sense of gratitude.**
   Even before saying the intention, get a sense of what you are grateful for in your life and what you have already accomplished. This is the most fertile soil in which to plant the seeds of your desires.

◆ **Inquire into any old memories that may override your intention.**

◆ **When setting an intention, always say it in the present time.**
   This will give the brain the message that your intention is already happening. Then, the energy follows the thought and like a magnet, you get what you desire.

Say *'I am'*, not *'I will'*

Say *'I have'*, not *'I want'*

◆ **Keep your intention simple, to the point and think big.**
   Often you can be caught in the details of a certain situation and limit yourself. Take a moment to see what the bigger picture is and ask for it all. Imagine your car needs some massive repairs and you are in a quandary over whether to spend a huge amount of money on the old car or to buy a new one. A good intention would be 'I have a reliable car that meets all my needs and is comfortably in my price range.' Then let the universe take care of how your intention is met, whether this is your old car being repaired or receiving the money or ability to buy a new one.

◆ **Say the intention often.**
   This will allow the intention to overlay and overpower any negative diminishing thoughts that may confuse or block you receiving the manifestation.

◈ **When setting an intention for yourself, make it heartfelt.**
This is your poignant communication line to the universe asking for the life you desire. Keep the intent clear, concise and simple to eliminate miscommunication.

Say it.
Know it.
Believe it.

"I remember years ago writing a very specific list for the man I desired to be in relationship with. Before long, he showed up in the perfect form apart from the one huge detail. He was gay and even though we became dear friends, it was obvious it would never be a romantic relationship. At the time, it never crossed my mind to put someone's sexual orientation into the mix. But now I do." ~ Miranda

SELF-INQUIRY

By gazing inward the true reflection of the self is revealed.

Remember, this inquiry is only between you and you. There is no one else here to judge. Also, let go of any of your own personal beliefs around who you think you *should* be. 'A Woman's Truth' is about no longer 'should-ing' all over yourself. As you reveal more of whom you truly are, it is vital you meet all these different aspects with love, even the parts of which you may not be so fond. The gentle persuasion of a loving attitude is much more influential in facilitating a change of heart.

Unveiling distortions is always the deepest and most valuable work you can do.

BE HONEST WITH YOURSELF, AS YOU LOOK INWARD:

◆ **What is most important to you in your life?**
You may prioritize your list if you have more than one idea. Some examples could be your health, your child, your sanity, your relationships, your security, being of service, making money, your job, your partner, your pets or your spiritual life.

◆ **What do you do freely and willingly on a daily basis?**

◆ Why do you do these activities?

◆ What do they provide for you?

◆ What do you desire to gain from your commitment to 'A Woman's Truth'?
When deciding on an intention for yourself, another way of asking this question is: 'What would enable me to live the fullest and most joyful life possible?'

◆ **What are the motivations behind these intentions?**
In other words, why do you want this for yourself?

◆ **What obstacles hinder the necessary actions to achieve your desires?**

◆ **What part of you do you need to lean into and make friends with in order to make this journey of transformation with compassion rather than judgment?**

◆ **What do you need to feel supported and to help keep the intention alive?**

what you cultivate, you will become.

WHAT LIES DO YOU LIVE BY?

Living your Truth.

What if you came into this world carrying with you three lies and until you became conscious of these falsehoods they would rule and influence your life? Who knows whether this is true or not, but you can achieve clarity by asking the simple question:

Can unveiling the lies that we live by
ultimately help reveal the truth?

The answer to this simple yet loaded question could ultimately help reveal your truths. As the lie is exposed, a new way of being can be implemented and your Truth can become the foundation of how you choose to live.

"I learned about this old belief of living by three lies years ago from a spiritual mentor. Something about it resonated with me, so I began an internal inquiry into what mine might be. The first lie that raised its head was my many distorted beliefs around my role as a healer. Through this journey, which lasted over a year, I let go of the very strong imprints that I had to heal people at all. This ultimately gave me a deep sense of freedom to be present with the extraordinary people I work with. Miraculously, I then seemed to be able to be more of a guiding light in their journey. This lie also involved the belief that to be loved I had to make people better and lastly that I was responsible for their healing, certainly a tall order! As you can imagine, a certain stress level went hand in hand with these beliefs. The second lie I uncovered was entangled in all the webs we weave about love. I feel I am still unraveling this one. And the third one...well it seems to be connected to giving too much power to the mind, instead of letting the mind be of service to the heart. This too is still a work in progress..." ~ Miranda

Interestingly these lies and deceptions can weave their way into the tapestry of your being. Yet, once revealed, it is as though the fabric unravels itself, exposing you to your Real Truth.

THEREFORE, THERE ARE TWO QUESTIONS TO ASK HERE:

◆ What lies do I live by?

◆ What then is my Truth?
Often this will be the opposite mirror to the lie.

SUCH A PERFECT DAY

Dream on...

Allow yourself to imagine what a perfect day would feel or be like for you. Every single aspect from waking to sleeping is absolutely what your heart desires. There would be no stress, no having to do anything. The day would ebb and flow with play, creativity, adventure, giving, receiving, rest, nourishment, and all-out doses of self-love.

what would this perfect day look like?

If you have not contemplated this question before, then it is high time this inquiry guided your imagination. Allow it to lead you into a world where earning money, doing chores, taking care of people and objects and the *to-do* list have no ground or power over you. Imagine a world where you are given the freedom to dream and actually see your ideal life, without all the veils of what you should be doing.

Obviously, if you are exhausted, a day at the spa or in bed will probably seem highly appealing. Take note of this. If rest is all you can think about, it is time for some serious self-care and a few pajama days in your life. If you are feeling exhausted or overwhelmed, then imagine a whole month of uninterrupted sleep, pampering, quiet, someone cooking for you, a personal trainer and all chores being taken care of, obviously not by you! Once you can imagine yourself replenished, then ask the question again.

Eventually you will get bored of doing nothing, honestly! There is an expression that says that you should never make a decision the day before your period. In translation, this means that it is always better to be balanced and centered before making any big, life-altering changes such as seeking the life you truly desire. If a perfect day feels too tight and limiting, imagine a perfect week or month instead.

GIVE YOURSELF SOME TIME TO PONDER
AND INQUIRE INTO YOUR PERFECT LIFE:

◆ What time would you go to bed and wake up?

◆ Is this day completely different to the next?

◆ How much down time do you desire?

◆ What would you do during this down time?

◆ How would you move the body?

◆ From where does your food appear or would you want to cook it yourself?

◆ Are you in the city, in nature or a mixture of both?

◆ Does your perfect day or week involve children, animals or socializing?

◆ What does the timeline look like if there is one?

◆ What job would you look forward to doing?

◈ How long would you want your workday to be?

◈ Would you want to drive somewhere and get out of the house or stay home?

◈ Would you spend time creating?

◈ What would you do for adventure?

◈ How much time alone would you enjoy?

◆ How do you nurture and nourish yourself?

◆ What else would make your life more perfect?

Allow your imagination to go wild.

Notice the voice that will keep telling you: 'It is not possible. Who is going to really take care of everything?' Thank this voice and remind yourself, this is all about becoming a visionary. Your rational and survival brain will not be able to go on this fantastic journey of imagination. So for now, leave her behind to worry over dinner and the bills. It is your imagination that will soar with this visualization. Play with your ideals and laugh at the limitations of your mundane life. This really is about allowing yourself to dream and to get a glimpse of the life you truly desire to live.

Literally, dream on...

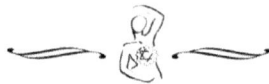

*"Laugh as much as you breathe
and love as long as you live."*

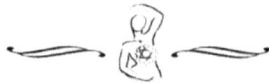

REVEAL MORE TRUTH

You have to do your own growing,
no matter how tall your grandmother was.

First, I want to thank you from my heart for your choice to commit to yourself. Every time a commitment is made and followed through, no matter how small, trust is built. I am sincerely grateful to you for undertaking this journey of falling in love with yourself and for sharing from your heart the innate and extraordinary wisdom inherent in you.

THE FOLLOWING ARE SIMPLE INVITATIONS
TO YOUR COMMITMENT TO LOVE YOURSELF:

◆ **Read through the writings in this book.**
Read a chapter a day or you can curl up with a cup of tea and go cover to cover. Either way, it is imperative to connect to these teachings daily as this practice will deepen your experience, support you and be a reminder of who you truly are.

◆ **Review the Obstacle List.**
Please prioritize five to ten of the obstacles that stand in the way of you taking exquisite care of yourself. Label number one being the biggest dam blocker. Spend some time inquiring whether this obstacle is actually a truth or not.

◆ **Review the questionnaire.**
Go through the questionnaire and highlight which of your habits are beneficial and which behaviors could do with some serious refining. Choose to replace one harmful habit with a more valuable one.

◆ **Answer the questions from the Self-Inquiry.**
This will help guide you to figure out your intention. It will give you clarity around what goals resonate with you and will facilitate the changes you desire.

◆ Write out a clear and loving intention for yourself.
  Remember, it can always change. Repeat this daily to strengthen your resolve.

◆ Inquire into what lies you may be living by.
  In my own experience, this is a lifelong question...

◆ Most importantly, choose to take exquisite and loving care of yourself.

I send abundant blessings to you for your participation and willingness to change. Transformation is a courageous act. I look forward to connecting with you again in the next chapter of your life as we explore 'The Grandeur of Sleep' and reveal the gift of rest and rejuvenation to you.

Sending you my love and support on this priceless journey,

Miranda

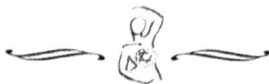

"Life is change.
Growth is optional.
Choose wisely."

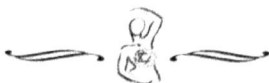

ABOUT MIRANDA

A spirited guide and mentor.

Miranda is a passionate and devoted leader. Her loving and wise support will guide you on a transformational journey as her powerful teachings unveil the truth of who you are. Her gift is to offer potent tools, which inspire exquisite and beautiful self-care and empower you to live the fullest and most authentic life possible. As a mentor and guide, Miranda deeply walks her talk and is fearless about her own path of self-discovery, as she weaves the sacred into the mundane.

The simple, yet powerful premise offered by the mystic Rumi is the foundation of Miranda's philosophy and mission:

"Never give from the depths of your well,
always give from your overflow."

Miranda gives Council and Guidance for the Mind, Body and Spirit. With a background in Nutrition and Energy work, Miranda is the Creator of 'A Woman's Truth' and 'The Spirit of Energy', an Author, a Workshop and Retreat Leader, a Reiki Master and Yoga and Meditation teacher. Miranda studies under the guidance of her Beloved teachers Rod Stryker and Adyashanti.

To speak with or follow Miranda, please call or visit:

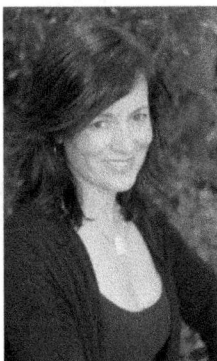

Phone: 626~798~6544
eMail: Info@MirandaJBarrett.com
Website: www.MirandaJBarrett.com
Facebook: Miranda J Barrett
Twitter: MirandaJBarrett

ABOUT HELENA

A visionary artist.

Helena Nelson-Reed is a visionary artist whose primary medium is watercolor. Born in Seattle, Washington, she was raised in Marin County and Napa Valley, California and today lives in Illinois. A largely self-taught artist whose educational emphasis and degree is in psychology, Nelson-Reed's primary focus is exploring the collective consciousness and the portrayal of archetypal imagery in the tradition of Carl Jung and Joseph Campbell. Rendered in luminous watercolor technique often described as ephemeral, Nelson-Reed's paintings are created in extraordinary detail, pushing the medium of watercolor past the usual limits. Her work may be found in private collections, book covers, magazines and CD covers. Nelson-Reed also has a line of jewelry, calendars and greeting cards.

Helena's Mission:

My images can be interpreted many ways, and for some they will serve as portal to the mythic landscape. Descriptions providing background about each painting are available by request. Navigating and translating myth into contemporary wisdom is the traditional way of transmitting information, a shamanic and multi - cultural practice.

Myth, fairy, folk and spiritual lore describe divine beings and supernatural life forms arriving unbidden and disguised. In our earthly dimension, mortals often play similar roles in the lives of one another. Destinies and energies collide and interact, visible and invisible forces are at work. The mythic realms are timeless, offering insight and inspiration. While my paintings have a positive energy, many have roots in the shadows of life experience and human psyche, as the lotus blossom rooted in pond mud. For many, life is one challenge followed by the next, like beads on an endless string.

Take heart! Like goddess Inanna, one may navigate the underworld, move through dark places yet return to the realms of light battle scarred but wiser, richer for the experience. Read the ancient tales, the great mythic literature; draw strength, for they are repositories of wisdom.

Visit Helena's website for her art purchase information and art to wear jewelry:

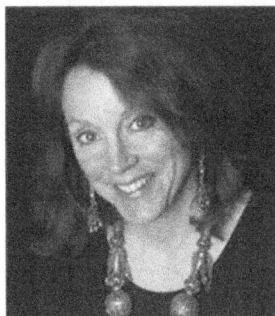

eMail: HNelsonReed@Gmail.com
Websites: www.HelenaNelsonReed.com
www.etsy.com/shop/HelenaNelsonReed
Blog: www.dancingdovestudio.blogspot.com
Facebook: MorningDove Design By Helena

MIRANDA'S WORLD

*Ways to stay connected
and aligned with your truth.*

BOOKS:

A Woman's Truth

A life truly worth living.

Priceless teachings reveal your transformational
journey ahead. Obstacles to self-care are explored
as clear and loving intentions are conceived.

The Grandeur Of Sleep

Permission to rest.

Miraculous benefits are realized as the worlds of sleep,
relaxation and rejuvenation are explored and deeply honored.

Nourishing Nutrition

Reclaim your health and vitality.

Reap the bountiful rewards while eating as nature intended.
Claim your health and vitality with these simple,
yet powerful tools to nourish and heal your body.

Embodying Movement
Ground your whole being.

Restore balance in your life. Discover how to embrace
your whole being through the life-enhancing benefits of body movement.

Body Care
Cherish your body as a temple.

Learn to honor your extraordinary body
as a living temple and listen to the healing messages she whispers.

Feminine Power
Fully access your supreme birthright.

Welcome and reclaim this intrinsic privilege while living
in harmonious balance between the masculine and the feminine.

The Abundance Of Wealth
Receive the gifts of prosperity.

Understand the energy flow of prosperity and weave
the threads of abundance throughout the tapestry of your life.

Find Your Authentic Voice
The courage to express who you truly are.

Your greatest ally is born
when you courageously speak your truth and claim your unique power.

Loving Yourself
A love affair with the self.

As you become highly attuned to your own needs,
allow love to lead the way. Grant yourself permission
to honor and express your heart's truest desires.
Love yourself, no matter what.

Living A Spiritual Life
Ground your divine essence here on earth.

Discover what spirituality means to you, by consciously
living between the two worlds of the sacred and the mundane.

Service As A Way of Life
Ignite the fire of love to truly be of service.

By utilizing the gems of exquisite self-care
on a daily basis and honoring your truth, your mission of service is born.

The Crowning Glory
Fully Rejoice in Being You.

A celebration overflowing with love,
blessings, grace and gratitude. Stand confident within
your truth as your mind begins to serve your heart.

The Food Of Life
The versatile vegetable.

More than just a cookbook,
a comprehensive guide for nourishing your life.

Reiki
The spirit of Energy.

An insightful guidebook full of wisdom
which introduces you to the potent and healing world of Reiki.

CARDS:

Inspiration Cards
A daily Spiritual Practice.

Sixty-Five cards with simple yet inspirational qualities
to live by and an insightful guidebook to lead the way.

CD'S:

The Grandeur of Sleep
and Rejuvenating Rest

An ancient healing art of rest and relaxation.

Simple yet profound practices that alleviate stress and tension
allowing your mind, body and spirit to heal, restore and replenish.

TO ORDER PLEASE VISIT:

www.MirandaJBarrett.com
www.Amazon.com

* All books are available in printed or eBook form.

TESTIMONIES

to 'A Woman's Truth' teachings

"If you're a woman, 'A Woman's Truth' is a must. Never have I received such a wealth of information in such a clear, concise and meaningful way. I remember taking my son home from the hospital thinking, "What, no Owner's Manual? No instructions?" This book is like an Owner's Manual for your life. Miranda provides you with the tools to achieve everything you desire in a safe, loving environment."

Diane ~ Business Consultant and Mother ~ Altadena, CA

"These teachings are the Queen in daily life, lovely, Divine and generous. Miranda's expertise, mastery and her loving delivery was exquisite. I gained a deeper commitment to self-care and it is no longer a mystery to me. I now love to take great care of myself and I have more love for myself and others; so much more than I knew was possible."

Shadee ~ PAX Workshop Leader ~ Marina Del Ray, CA

"Miranda has created a remarkable journey for women. I now treasure myself and have come to see how extremely important it is to take care of myself as a woman."

Valerie ~ Teacher and Dream Builder ~ Pasadena, CA

"The positive and loving framework throughout these books allowed me to explore myself and create an environment in my life to foster growth and self-care. It was a context that opened up new possibilities that I did not know existed and gave me the courage to pursue them. It was like a big hug that held me as I went out and explored the waters of self-care and femininity"

Kim ~ Dance Teacher ~ Glendale, CA

www.ingramcontent.com/pod-product-compliance
Lightning Source LLC
LaVergne TN
LVHW061229060426
835509LV00012B/1475